HEALT[ ]
RECFIPES FOR
BEGINNERS

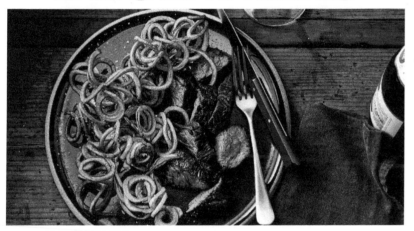

LUNCH

Paola Clifford

Welcome!

To this new series of book, inspired by all the recipes I know thanks to my great passion: *cooking!*

"You really know what you are eating if you make it yourself"

In this book you will find many different ideas for your dishes, with ingredients from all around the world, with a Gourmet touch!

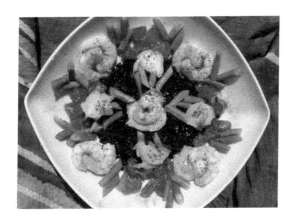

Thanks to these cookbooks you can develop your cooking skills for any kind of meal, as you'll find recipes for:

★ salads
★ sides
★ lunch
★ dinner
★ Desserts

And much more...

Whether your favourite dish is French fries, muffins, chicken tenders or grilled vegetables, with this series of books you will learn how to do it with a better-looking touch!

Don't forget that this books have also low fat recipes with healthy ingredients to *keep you fit and have a healthier meal plan!*

Remember that having a wide variety of ingredients and foods in your diet have many benefits for you, that's why you will find ingredients from:

- ★ Asia
- ★ Russia
- ★ America
- ★ Europe

And much more...

Since I started to pay more attention on the decision of the ingredients and how to plate a dish, I enjoy cooking a lot more! That's why I made this cookbook for all of you that want to develop your cooking skills and start eating healthier!

I hope you will enjoy this book! Don't forget to check out the other ones from the collection, and enjoy your time in the kitchen!

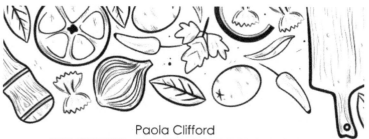

Paola Clifford

HEALTHY RECIPES
FOR BEGINNERS

LUNCH

LEARN HOW TO MIX DIFFERENT INGREDIENTS AND SPICES TO
CREATE DELICIOUS DISHES AND BUILD A COMPLETE MEAL PLAN!
THIS COOKBOOK INCLUDES QUICK RECIPES TO PREPARE ON A
DAILY BASIS, FOR AN EFFECTIVE DIET AND A HEALTHIER LIFESTYLE!

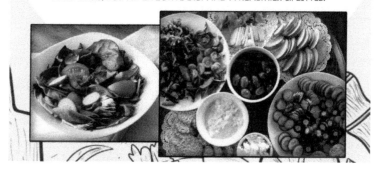

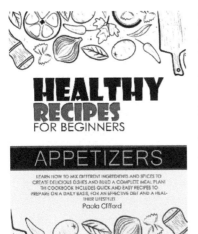

HEALTHY RECIPES FOR BEGINNERS: APPETIZERS

Learn how to mix different ingredients and spices to create delicious dishes and build a complete meal plan! This cookbook includes quick recipes to prepare on a daily basis, for an effective diet and a healthier lifestyle!

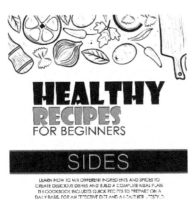

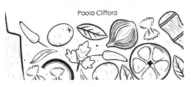

HEALTHY RECIPES FOR BEGINNERS: SIDES

Learn how to mix different ingredients and spices to create delicious dishes and build a complete meal plan! This cookbook includes quick recipes to prepare on a daily basis, for an effective diet and a healthier lifestyle!

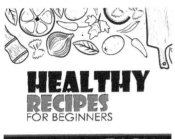

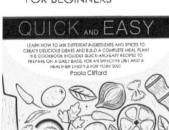

HEALTHY RECIPES FOR BEGINNERS: QUICK AND EASY

Learn how to mix different ingredients and spices to create delicious dishes and build a complete meal plan! This cookbook includes quick-and-easy recipes to prepare on a daily basis, for an effective diet and a Healthier lifestyle for your 2021!

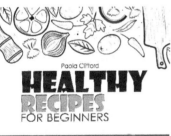

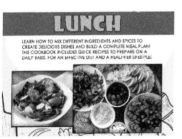

HEALTHY RECIPES FOR BEGINNERS: LUNCH

Learn how to mix different ingredients and spices to create delicious dishes and build a complete meal plan! This cookbook includes quick recipes to prepare on a daily basis, for an effective diet and a healthier lifestyle!

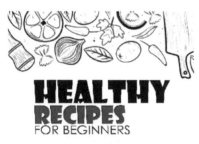

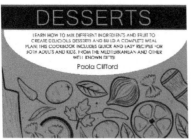

HEALTHY RECIPES FOR BEGINNERS: DESSERTS

Learn how to mix different ingredients and fruit to create delicious desserts and build a complete meal plan! This cookbook includes quick and easy recipes for both adults and kids, from the Mediterranean and other well-known diets!

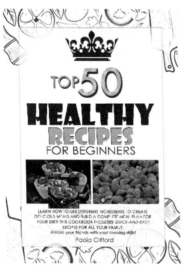

HEALTHY RECIPES FOR BEGINNERS: TOP 50

Learn how to mix different ingredients to create Delicious meals and build a complete meal plan for your diet! This cookbook includes quick-and-easy recipes for all your family. Amaze your friends with your cooking skills!

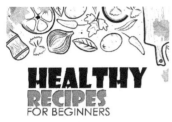

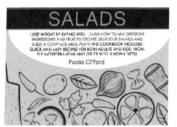

HEALTHY RECIPES FOR BEGINNERS: SALADS

Lose weight by eating well! Learn how to mix different ingredients and fruit to create delicious salads and build a complete meal plan! This cookbook includes quick and easy recipes for both adults and kids, from the mediterranean and other well-known diets!

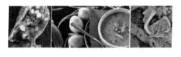

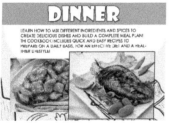

HEALTHY RECIPES FOR BEGINNERS: DINNER

Learn how to mix different ingredients and spices to create delicious dishes and build a complete meal plan! This cookbook includes quick and easy recipes to prepare on a daily basis, for an effective diet and a healthier lifestyle!

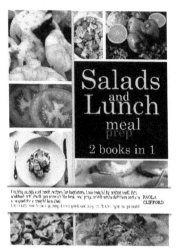

SALADS AND LUNCH MEAL PREP

2 books in 1: Healthy salad and lunch recipes for beginners. Lose weight by eating well! This cookbook contains some of the best low-fat recipes that also ideal for weight loss and body-healing routines. Improve your cooking skills with the right book!

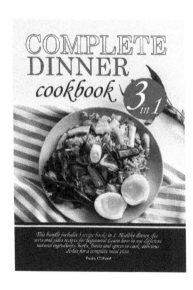

COMPLETE DINNER COOKBOOK

This boundle contains 3 recipe books in 1: healthy dinner, desserts and sides recipes for beginner.

Learn how to use different ingredients, herbs, spices and plants to cook delicious dishes for your complete meal plan.

Table of Contents

NOT YOUR USUAL LUNCH RECIPES

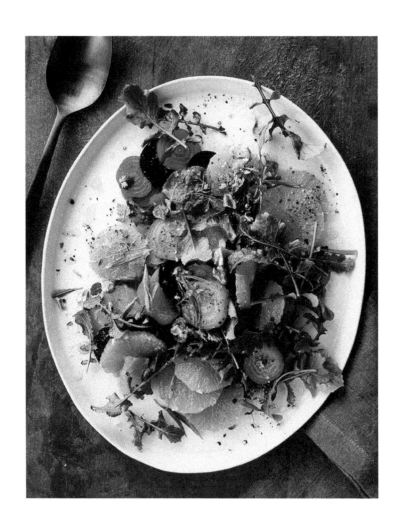

Gourmet Stuffed Pork Chops

Serving: 2

Ingredients

- 2 (3/4 inch thick) bone-in pork chops

- 1 (4 ounce) package sliced fresh mushrooms

- 4 ounces diced Swiss cheese

- 1 tablespoon chopped fresh parsley

- 1 teaspoon garlic powder

- 1/4 teaspoon ground black pepper

- 1/4 teaspoon salt

- 2 eggs

- 3/4 cup bread crumbs

- 2 tablespoons vegetable oil

- 1/2 cup white Zinfandel wine, or as needed

Direction

- Place the pork chop evenly on a work surface. Slice a 2-in slit on the side of each pork chop using the tip of a sharp paring or boning knife to form pockets.

- In a bowl, combine salt, mushrooms, black pepper, Swiss cheese, garlic powder, and parsley. Scoop the mushroom mixture into the pork chop pockets. Use a toothpick to seal the open sides.

- Beat eggs in a bowl. Put bread crumbs in another bowl. Submerge the stuffed pork chops in the whisked eggs and dredge in the bowl of bread crumbs until well covered.

- On medium heat, pour oil in a pan and heat. Put the pork chops pocket-side down in the heated oil. Cook for 2-3 minutes each side until the pork chops are brown on the outside.

- Pour in wine until the chops are covered halfway. Turn heat to low, cover the pan, and let it simmer for 2 hours until the pork chops are tender. Intermittently check the wine level and pour in more if required. An inserted thermometer in the middle of the pork should register 63°C or 145°F.

Nutrition Information

- Calories: 878 calories;

- Total Fat: 51.9

- Sodium: 813

- Total Carbohydrate: 36.2

- Cholesterol: 310

- Protein: 55.3

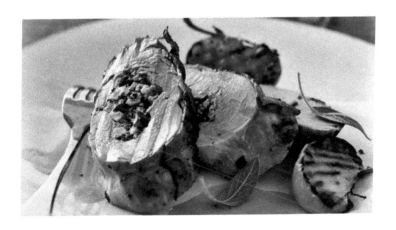

Grandma Me's Clove Studded Leg Of Lamb

Serving: 8

Ingredients

- 1 (6 pound) bone-in leg of lamb, trimmed

- 1 tablespoon whole cloves

- 1 (12 ounce) can apricot nectar

- 1 teaspoon salt

- 1 pinch black pepper

- 1/4 teaspoon soy sauce

- 4 slices lemon, for garnish

- 2 teaspoons cornstarch

- 1/2 cup water

- 1 cube vegetable bouillon, crushed

Direction

- Set oven to 165° C (325° F) and start preheating.

- Slice through the narrow end of lamb leg with a sharp knife, about 3 inches from the end. Slice through the meat surrounding the bone. Take out this piece and discard, keeping the clean exposed bone. (You can ask the butcher to do this for you.) Stick an even pattern of cloves into the lamb leg. Arrange in a metal shallow roasting pan.

- Place in the preheated oven and bake 2 hours. Drain to remove drippings and fat. In a small bowl, whisk together soy sauce, pepper, salt and apricot nectar; spread over lamb leg. Bring the lamb back to the oven and bake, basting often, until inserting a meat thermometer into the thickest part and it shows 71° C (160° F) for medium-well doneness. Place lemon slices atop the roast; bake 5 more minutes.

- Transfer lamb to a serving plate, use aluminum foil to cover. Let sit 10-15 minutes, then slice.

In the meantime, on the stove over medium heat, place the roasting pan. Put cornstarch in water and dissolve; add to the roasting pan together with the bouillon cube. Cook while stirring for 1 minutes until the sauce clears and thickens, and bouillon is dissolved. Take out lemon slices and cloves. Then slice the lamb and serve with sauce.

Nutrition Information

- Calories: 414 calories;

- Total Carbohydrate: 8

- Cholesterol: 138

- Protein: 38.3

- Total Fat: 24.6

- Sodium: 404

Grape, Chicken, And Walnut Pesto Pizza

Serving: 4

Ingredients

- 1 (16 ounce) package refrigerated pizza dough (such as Trader Joe's®)
- 1/4 cup prepared pesto (such as Classico®)
- 1 1/2 cups shredded mozzarella cheese
- 1/2 cup cooked shredded chicken
- 15 red seedless grapes, halved lengthwise
- 2 tablespoons walnut pieces
- ground black pepper to taste (optional)

Direction

- Set the oven to 350°F (175°C) and start preheating.

- Evenly spread pizza dough onto a pizza pan.

- Bake dough for about 8 minutes on preheated oven until cooked slightly.

- Spread a thin layer of pesto onto pizza crust, leaving edges exposed. Add mozzarella on top of pesto layer; add chicken. Place grapes around the crust, cut-side up. Add walnuts on top of pizza and add black pepper to season.

- Bake for about 10 minutes in preheated oven until crust's bottom is light brown in color and the cheese is melted.

Nutrition Information

- Calories: 550 calories;

- Cholesterol: 45

- Protein: 28.4

- Total Fat: 21.6

- Sodium: 1139

- Total Carbohydrate: 59.2

Greek Flank Steak

Serving: 4

Ingredients

1 flank steak

butcher's twine

salt and ground black pepper to taste

1 bunch baby spinach

1/4 cup crumbled feta cheese

1/4 cup chopped kalamata olives

2 strips cooked crispy bacon (optional)

Direction

- Set a charcoal griller (such as Big Green Egg®) at 175°C (375°F) to preheat and lightly grease the grate.

- On a flat surface, lay the flank steak. From 1 side of the steak, cut horizontally through the middle to within 1/2 inch of the other side. Open the 2 sides and spread them out like an open book.

- Arrange enough butcher's twine on a plate to cover the length of the steak. Set about 1-inch distance between each string. Then place the steak on top; season with pepper and salt. Lay down on top a thick bed of spinach. Spread bacon, olives, and feta cheese over the spinach.

- Roll up the steak beginning from the closest edge to you, pressing the filling down to tighten the roll. Use butcher's twine to tie.

- Cook over direct heat for 6 to 7 minutes per side, flipping for at least 1 time, until the steak starts to become hot, firm, and slightly pink in the center. An instant-read thermometer should read 140°F (60°C) when inserted into the center.

Nutrition Information

- Calories: 354 calories;

- Sodium: 676

- Total Carbohydrate: 4.4

- Cholesterol: 77

- Protein: 37.2

- Total Fat: 20.5

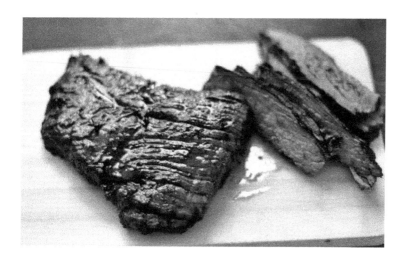

Bacon Trout

Serving: 4

Ingredients

- 1/4 cup butter

- 1 lemon, juiced

- 2 tablespoons seeded and diced jalapeno pepper

- 2 tablespoons diced green onion

- 1/2 clove garlic, minced

- sea salt and ground black pepper to taste

- 2 (10 ounce) cleaned whole trout, heads removed

- 2 sprigs fresh dill

- 2 slices bacon

Direction

- Set oven to 400°F (200°C) for preheating.

- Line a glass baking dish of 9x13 inches with foil.

- Heat butter in a small saucepan over low heat until melted partially. Mix in garlic, green onion, jalapeno pepper, lemon juice; stir mixture into a paste. Add sea salt and black pepper to season.

- Arrange each trout on a large sheet of aluminum foil then use butter paste to stuff the cavity of each fish; into the cavity while on top of the butter mixture, place a dill sprig and bacon strip. Fold foil over fish and wrap edges to seal tightly. Put foil packets in the prepared baking dish.

- Let foil packets bake for 26 minutes, until fish is easily flaked with a fork. Leave the fish to rest in foil packet for 5 minutes before removing the aluminum foil. Serve fish on serving a plate from foil; remove bacon. The fish's flesh would be white and skin would peel off.

Nutrition Information

- Calories: 295 calories;

- Total Fat: 18.3

- Sodium: 310

- Total Carbohydrate: 0.6

- Cholesterol: 118

- Protein: 30.6

Grilled Asparagus Steak Bundles

Serving: 2

Ingredients

- 1/2 pound thin skirt steak, trimmed of excess fat

- 1 tablespoon Montreal steak seasoning

- 1/2 pound thin asparagus spears, trimmed

- 1 teaspoon olive oil

- salt and ground black pepper to taste

- 1/3 cup grated Parmesan cheese

- 1/2 jarred roasted red pepper, cut into six 1/2-inch strips

- 6 toothpicks

- 1 tablespoon grated Parmesan cheese, or to taste

Direction

Beat steak using a meat mallet or butterfly to 1/4-inch thick. Slice in six 2" wide by 5" long strips. Season each strip on both sides using Montreal steak seasoning then refrigerate.

Set Countertop Induction Oven on medium high using the Grill setting.

Put asparagus in a short-sided dish then on top sprinkle olive oil. Sprinkle with salt and pepper to season.

Cook asparagus on grill for 2 minutes, turning once after a minute, then put on a plate.

Heat oven again on medium high using the Grill setting.

Position the steak strips next to each other in a line. Sprinkle 1/3 cup of parmesan cheese evenly over strips. Put 3-4 asparagus spears over them, perpendicular to every strip. Put 1 red pepper strip on every asparagus.

Roll steak around the asparagus tightly. Angle diagonally to not overlap the steak. Use toothpicks to secure.

Let steak bundles cook on the grill 8 minutes, flipping every 2 minutes. Put cooked steak bundles on a plate then drizzle on a tablespoon of parmesan cheese before serving.

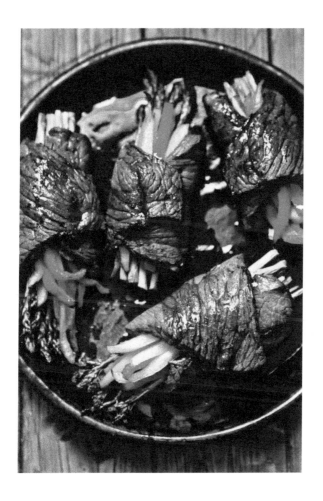

Grilled Cornish Game Hens

Serving: 4

Ingredients

1/2 onion, chopped

2 cloves garlic, peeled and chopped

1 cup lemon juice

1/2 cup olive oil

1 tablespoon white wine

1 teaspoon Worcestershire sauce

1 teaspoon hot pepper sauce

1 tablespoon pepper

1 teaspoon celery salt

1 teaspoon salt

4 (1 1/2 pound) Cornish game hens

Direction

Combine salt, celery salt, pepper, hot pepper sauce, Worcestershire sauce, white wine, olive oil, lemon juice, garlic, and onion in a large non-reactive bowl. In the bowl, arrange Cornish game hens and coat them evenly with marinade mixture. Put on a cover and put in the fridge to marinate for at least 4 hours.

Set an outdoor grill for medium heat and start preheating, then lightly brush grate with oil.

On the preheated grill, cook the hens for an hour, brushing with the remaining marinade from time to time until juices from hens run clear and hens are not pink anymore.

Nutrition Information

Calories: 871 calories;

Protein: 52.1

Total Fat: 69.2

Sodium: 1124

Total Carbohydrate: 8.5

Cholesterol: 302

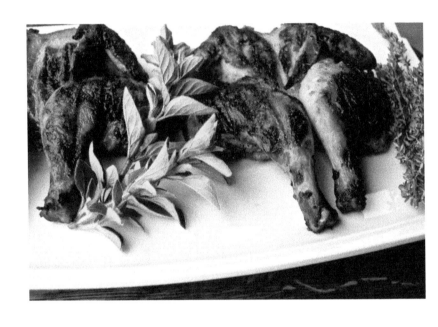

Grilled Fish Steaks

Serving: 8

Ingredients

8 (3 ounce) fillets fresh tuna steaks, 1 inch thick

1/2 cup soy sauce

1/3 cup sherry

1/4 cup vegetable oil

1 tablespoon fresh lime juice

1 clove garlic, minced

Direction

In a shallow baking dish, put in the tuna steaks. Combine the vegetable oil, soy sauce, fresh lime juice, garlic and sherry in a medium-sized bowl. Coat all sides of the tuna steaks with the soy sauce mixture. Cover the tuna steaks and keep in the fridge for at least an hour.

Preheat the grill to high heat.

Slightly grease the grill grate with oil. Put the marinated tuna steaks on the grill without the marinade. Cook the tuna steaks on the grill for 3-6 minutes each side until the desired doneness is achieved.

Nutrition Information

Calories: 171 calories;

Total Fat: 7.6

Sodium: 993

Total Carbohydrate: 3

Cholesterol: 38

Protein: 20.9

Grilled Lime Cilantro Ahi With Honey Glaze

Serving: 4 |

Ingredients

- 1/4 cup olive oil

- 1/4 cup lime juice

- 1/8 cup balsamic vinegar

- 2 cloves garlic, minced

- 1 tablespoon minced fresh ginger root

- 1/4 cup chopped cilantro

- 1 pound yellowfin tuna fillets

- 1/4 cup honey

- 2 tablespoons olive oil

- 2 tablespoons chopped cilantro

Direction

Combine 1/4 cup of cilantro, ginger, garlic, balsamic vinegar, lime juice, and 1/4 cup of olive oil in a medium-sized bowl. Add tuna fillets, flip to cover evenly. Put in the fridge to marinate for a few hours.

Set an outdoor grill to high heat and start preheating. Use oil to lightly grease the grate. Combine 2 tablespoons of cilantro, 2 tablespoons of olive oil, and honey in a small bowl. Put aside.

Once the grill is heated, lower the heat to low and put the tuna fillets on the grate. Shut the lid and cook for 1-2 minutes. Gently turn the fillets over and shut the lid again for an addition of 1 minute to sear the fish. Open the lid and keep cooking until barely done, use the marinade to frequently baste. Once the fish is nearly done, brush both sides of the fish with honey glaze and take away from the grill.

Nutrition Information

Calories: 379 calories;

Sodium: 48

Total Carbohydrate: 20.8

Cholesterol: 51

Protein: 26.9

Total Fat: 21.4

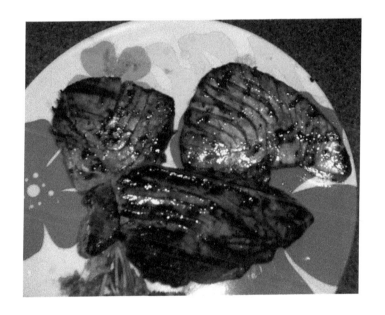

Grilled Salmon With Avocado Dip

Serving: 6

Ingredients

2 avocados - peeled, pitted and diced

2 cloves garlic, peeled and minced

3 tablespoons Greek-style yogurt

1 tablespoon fresh lemon juice

salt and pepper to taste

2 pounds salmon steaks

2 teaspoons dried dill weed

2 teaspoons lemon pepper

salt to taste

Direction

Prepare an outdoor grill by preheating to high and put oil on the grate lightly.

Mash together in a medium bowl the lemon juice, yogurt, garlic and avocados. Add pepper and salt to taste.

Then rub salmon with salt, lemon pepper and dill. Put on the preheated grill and cook for 15 minutes, flipping once, until easily flaked with fork. Then serve with the avocado mixture.

Nutrition Information

Calories: 396 calories;

Cholesterol: 91

Protein: 32

Total Fat: 26.9

Sodium: 640

Total Carbohydrate: 6.8

Grilled Shrimp Rice Noodle Bowl

Serving: 2

Ingredients

- 8 large fresh shrimp, peeled and deveined
- 3 tablespoons olive oil
- 3 cloves garlic
- 1/2 cup fresh mint
- 1/4 cup chopped fresh cilantro
- 3 tablespoons fish sauce
- 2 tablespoons honey
- 1 lime, juiced
- 1/4 teaspoon ground white pepper
- 2 tablespoons fresh ginger root, minced
- 3/4 cup shredded cabbage

- 1 (6.75 ounce) package dried rice noodles

Direction

- Heat grill for high heat. Mix white pepper, lime juice, honey, fish sauce, cilantro, 1/4 cup of mint, and garlic in a blender or food processor. Puree it until smooth.

- Boil a big pot of water. Cook cabbage and noodles until done for 2 minutes.

- As it cooks, use olive oil to coat shrimp then grill on high heat, flipping once, until golden.

- Mince leftover 1/4 cup of mint. Serve cabbage and noodles inside a bowl. Top with shrimp and sauce. Sprinkle with mint.

Nutrition Information

- Calories: 565 calories;

- Total Fat: 21.3

- Sodium: 1757

- Total Carbohydrate: 85

- Cholesterol: 44

- Protein: 10

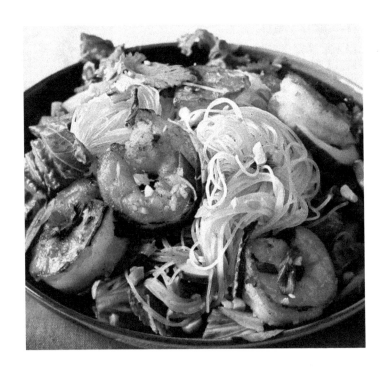

Grilled Stuffed Swordfish

Serving: 6

Ingredients

- 1 1/2 pounds swordfish steaks
- 1/4 cup dry white wine
- 1/4 cup soy sauce
- 1 tablespoon prepared Dijon-style mustard
- 1 teaspoon grated fresh ginger root
- 2 cloves garlic, minced
- 1 teaspoon sesame oil
- 3 tablespoons olive oil
- 1/4 cup fresh lemon juice
- 4 cups coarsely chopped arugula
- 3 tablespoons olive oil
- 3 tablespoons lemon juice

- 1 cup chopped fresh tomato

Direction

- Wash the swordfish well and pat to dry. Place the fish in a glass baking dish. Mix mustard, sesame oil, a 1/4 cup of lemon juice, olive oil, white wine, garlic, ginger, and soy sauce in a large mixing bowl. Drizzle sauce all over the fish. Cover the dish and store it inside the fridge for several hours or overnight.

- Get the swordfish and reserve its marinade. Cut pockets into the sides of the swordfish steaks using a sharp knife.

- Toss tomato, 3 tbsp. lemon juice, 3 tbsp. of olive oil, and arugula in a large bowl. Stuff arugula mixture into the swordfish and seal it with toothpicks.

- In a small saucepan, cook the marinade over high heat until the liquid is reduced by half.

- Preheat a grill or broiler to high heat. Grill each side of the swordfish for 5 minutes. Before serving, spoon the reduced marinade all over the swordfish.

Nutrition Information

- Calories: 296 calories;

- Sodium: 763

- Total Carbohydrate: 5.8

- Cholesterol: 44

- Protein: 23.7

- Total Fat: 19

Grilled Swordfish With Rosemary

Serving: 4

Ingredients

- 1/2 cup white wine

- 5 cloves garlic, minced

- 2 teaspoons chopped fresh rosemary

- 4 (4 ounce) swordfish steaks

- 1/4 teaspoon salt

- 1/4 teaspoon ground black pepper

- 2 tablespoons lemon juice

- 1 tablespoon extra virgin olive oil

- 4 slices lemon, for garnish

Direction

- In an 8-inch square baking dish, mix 1 tsp. of rosemary, garlic, and wine. Season the fish with pepper and salt, and then arrange it into the baking dish, flipping until coated. Cover the dish and place it inside the fridge for at least 1 hour.

- Mix olive oil, remaining rosemary, and lemon juice in a small bowl. Put the mixture aside.

- Set the grill to medium heat for preheating.

- Line the dish with paper towel. Transfer the fish onto the prepared dish, discarding the marinade. To prevent it from sticking, lightly coat oil onto the grill grate. Grill the fish for 10 minutes, flipping it only once, or until it can be flaked easily with a fork. Transfer the fish to a serving plate. Drizzle fish with lemon sauce. Garnish the top of each fillet with a lemon slice.

Nutrition Information

- Calories: 202 calories;

- Sodium: 248

- Total Carbohydrate: 4.3

- Cholesterol: 44

- Protein: 22.6

- Total Fat: 7.9

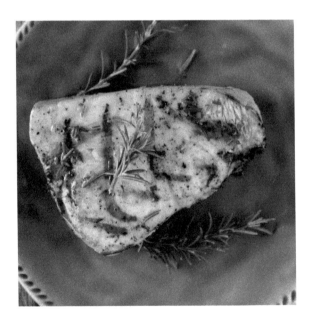

Grilled Turkey Breast With Fresh Sage Leaves

Serving: 8

Ingredients

- 3 tablespoons freshly squeezed lemon juice

- 3 tablespoons extra-virgin olive oil

- 28 leaves fresh sage

- 4 skinless, boneless turkey breast halves

- sea salt and freshly ground black pepper to taste

- 2 tablespoons extra-virgin olive oil

- 3 tablespoons unsalted butter

- 2 lemons, halved

Direction

- Combine 3 tablespoons olive oil, sage leaves, and lemon juice in a big container, mix them together and put the turkey breast halves into the mixture. Marinate the breasts at room temperature for 30 minutes and occasionally turn over the meat.

- Prepare the grill by preheating it to medium heat then coat the grate lightly with oil.

- Take the turkey breasts out of the marinade and set the marinade and sage leaves aside.

- Dash with sea salt and black pepper on both sides of the turkey.

- Cook the turkey breasts on the grill for about 30 minutes until grill marks appear, the inside of the meat is no longer pink and an instant-read meat thermometer reads at least 160° F (70° C) when inserted into the thickest part of the turkey breast. Flip over the turkey pieces after 15 minutes.

- Heat 2 tablespoons olive oil mixed with unsalted butter in a large pan on medium high-heat until hot and bubbles form, while the turkey is grilling. Add the marinate and the sage that you've set aside, into the oil and butter and continue cooking and stirring for 10 to 15 minutes until the marinade completely evaporates and the sage leaves are fried to crispiness.

- Move the grilled meat to a cutting board and add salt and black pepper, seasoning if you prefer; cut the turkey in diagonal thick slices and arrange the slices on a plate. Top the turkey slices with fried sage leaves and put lemon halves for garnish.

Nutrition Information

- Calories: 377 calories;

- Total Carbohydrate: 3.8

- Cholesterol: 168

- Protein: 57.1

- Total Fat: 14.3

- Sodium: 139

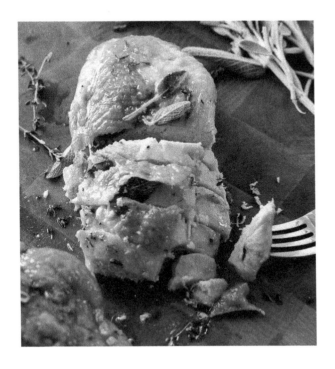

Ground Chicken With Walnuts

Serving: 10

Ingredients

- 1 (4 pound) chicken, cut into pieces

- 1 medium whole potato, peeled

- 1 small whole onion, peeled

- 1 small whole carrot, peeled

- 4 cups water

- 1 1/2 teaspoons salt

- 2 (1 inch thick) slices stale French bread, crusts removed

- 14 ounces walnuts, ground

- 2 cloves garlic, crushed

- 2 teaspoons ground red pepper

- 1 teaspoon salt

Direction

Put into a big saucepan with carrot, onion, potato and chicken on moderate heat. Add in water then bring to a boil. Skim any foam floating on the surface and use 1 1/2 tsp. of salt to season. Lower heat and simmer for an hour, until both vegetables and chicken are softened. Strain broth and reserve. Get rid of vegetables. Let chicken cool, then take off both skin and bones and shred the meat into extremely small pieces.

In some of the chicken broth, soften bread and then squeeze them out. Mix together 1 tsp. of salt, red pepper, garlic, ground walnuts and bread in a big bowl. Mix well with your hands like mixing meatballs. Put the mixture in cheesecloth and squeeze oil that the ground walnuts generate into a small bowl, then put aside. Put walnut mixture in a big bowl. Blend in 1 cup of reserved chicken broth gradually until you get a thick soup consistency.

In a porcelain or glass serving dish, add shredded chicken, stir in 2-3 tbsp. of walnut mixture. Use leftover walnut mixture to cover chicken so it is invisible. Use the back of a spoon to level the surface. Drizzle over top with reserved walnut oil.

Nutrition Information

- Calories: 691 calories;

- Cholesterol: 136

- Protein: 41.2

- Total Fat: 53.4

- Sodium: 754

- Total Carbohydrate: 14.1

Herb Crusted Halibut

Serving: 4

Ingredients

- 3/4 cup panko bread crumbs
- 1/3 cup chopped fresh parsley
- 1/4 cup chopped fresh dill
- 1/4 cup chopped fresh chives
- 1 tablespoon extra-virgin olive oil
- 1 teaspoon finely grated lemon zest
- 1 teaspoon sea salt
- 1/4 teaspoon ground black pepper
- 4 (6 ounce) halibut fillets

Direction

- Preheat an oven to 200°C/400°F.
- Line foil on a baking sheet.

- In a bowl, mix black pepper, sea salt, lemon zest, extra-virgin olive oil, chives, dill, parsley and panko breadcrumbs. Taste then adjust with extra salt if needed.

- Rinse the halibut flakes. Use a paper towel to pat dry.

- In prepped baking sheet, put halibut fillets.

- Spoon herbed crumbs generously on fish. Press crumb mixture lightly on every fillet.

- In preheated oven, bake for 10-15 minutes till fish easily flakes with a fork and crumb topping is browned lightly.

Nutrition Information

- Calories: 273 calories;

- Total Fat: 7.2

- Sodium: 778

- Total Carbohydrate: 14.8

- Cholesterol: 62

- Protein: 38.3

Herbed Pork And Apples

Serving: 14

Ingredients

- 1 teaspoon dried sage

- 1 teaspoon dried thyme

- 1 teaspoon dried rosemary

- 1 teaspoon dried marjoram

- salt and pepper to taste

- 6 pounds pork loin roast

- 4 tart apples - peeled, cored, cut into 1 inch chunks

- 1 red onion, chopped

- 3 tablespoons brown sugar

- 1 cup apple juice

- 2/3 cup real maple syrup

Direction

- Combine pepper, salt, marjoram, rosemary, thyme, and sage in a small bowl. Rub mixture all over roast. Chill, covered, for 6 to 8 hours or overnight.

- Turn oven to 325°F (165°C) to preheat.

- Positon roast in a shallow roasting pan; bake for 60 to 90 minutes in the preheated oven. Drain fat.

- Mix onion and apples with brown sugar in a medium bowl. Spread around roast; keep baking until a temperature registers 145°F (63°C), for 60 minutes longer. Remove roast, onion, and apples to a serving platter and keep warm.

- For gravy: ladle fat off the pan juices. Transfer drippings into a medium heavy skillet, mix in syrup and apple juice. Cook over medium-high heat, stirring often, until liquid is reduced by 1/2 (or about 1 cup). Serve roast in slices with gravy.

Nutrition Information

- Calories: 358 calories;

- Total Fat: 21.1

- Sodium: 29

- Total Carbohydrate: 21.3

- Cholesterol: 79

- Protein: 20.4

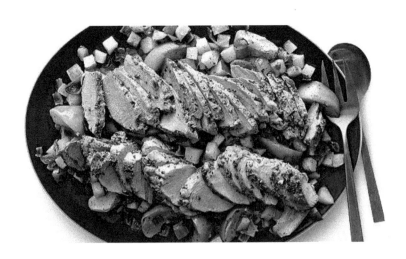

Homemade Chorizo

Serving: 8

Ingredients

- 1 clove garlic

- 3 teaspoons dried oregano

- 1/2 cup distilled white vinegar

- 1/2 cup crushed red pepper flakes

- 1/2 cup water

- 2 1/2 pounds ground pork

Direction

- Combine water, red pepper flakes, vinegar, oregano and garlic in a blender. Blend until they become smooth.

- Pour the mixture in a bowl over the ground pork. Place in the refrigerator with a cover all day. Remove all the water that accumulates.

Place in the refrigerator or freezer for other use.

Nutrition Information

- Calories: 322 calories;

- Sodium: 75

- Total Carbohydrate: 5.5

- Cholesterol: 92

- Protein: 26.3

- Total Fat: 21.9

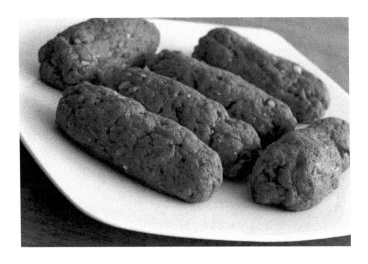

Homemade Pear And Gorgonzola Ravioli

Serving: 4

Ingredients

- 3 tablespoons butter
- 2 ripe pears - peeled, cored, and cubed
- 3 sprigs fresh thyme
- 7 ounces Gorgonzola cheese, crumbled
- 1 pound fresh pasta dough

Direction

In a big skillet, melt butter over medium heat. Put in thyme and pears; cook for 10 minutes, mixing frequently, till pears have softened. Crumble Gorgonzola cheese on top of pears; cook and mix for 2 to 3 minutes till melted. Take off skillet from heat and cool filling fully.

Slice pasta dough into 3 even pieces. On a floured work surface, flatten the first piece of dough; roll using a rolling pin for 5 or 6 times. Turn the dough 45 degrees and roll once more, 5 to 6 times. Continue rolling and turning in the same direction till dough has a consistent thickness of approximately 1/16-inch. Redo with leftover 2 pieces of pasta dough.

On a floured surface, slowly put 1 pasta sheet and halve to create 2 equally sized rectangles. Drop 1 teaspoon filling onto 1 rectangle, spacing the filling about 1-inch apart. Brush the spaces surrounding the filling with water.

Put the second rectangle over the first. Slowly press out the air around the filling and pinch firmly with your hands to secure the edges and all the dough around the filling.

Cut ravioli in square forms with a ravioli cutter. Put the ravioli onto a floured board or plate. Redo with the rest of the dough and filling. Allow the ravioli to stand for half an hour.

Boil a saucepan of lightly salted water; in batches, slowly add ravioli. Cook for 3 minutes till ravioli float to the top. Take out with a slotted spoon and put into a warm bowl.

Nutrition Information

- Calories: 555 calories;

- Total Fat: 24.8

- Sodium: 569

- Total Carbohydrate: 62.3

- Cholesterol: 80

- Protein: 20.8

Italian Style Pork Tenderloin

Serving: 4

Ingredients

3 1/2 pounds pork tenderloin

2 cloves garlic, minced

15 oil-cured black olives, pitted

1 teaspoon prepared mustard

salt and pepper to taste

1 red bell pepper, halved and deseeded

4 fresh mushrooms

1 onion, thinly sliced

1 tablespoon browning sauce

Direction

Slice and spread the pork tenderloin open the long way. Place the minced garlic, chopped olives, and mustard into the roast. Sprinkle all over the roast with salt and pepper to taste. Shape the loin into a roll and tie it securely with 1-inch intervals. Refrigerate the tenderloin and marinate for 24 hours.

In grilling the pork, set the grill to high heat.

Place the sliced red pepper on the bottom of the heavy-duty foil. Top the pepper with the marinated tenderloin. Paint the tenderloin with the browning sauce. Top it with mushrooms and onion slices. Seal the foil, making sure that there's a little tent on top.

Grill the pork in the grill for 20 minutes until its internal temperature reaches 145°F (63°C). Remove it from the heat and allow the pork to rest for 10 minutes before slicing it.

In baking the pork, set the oven to 375°F (190°C) for preheating.

Arrange the sliced red pepper onto the roasting pan's bottom. Top the pepper with the marinated tenderloin.

Paint the surface with the browning sauce. Top it with mushrooms and onion slices. Cover the pan and bake it inside the preheated oven for 30 minutes until its internal temperature reaches 145°F (63°C). Allow the pork to rest for 10 minutes before carving it.

Nutrition Information

Calories: 532 calories;

Cholesterol: 258

Protein: 83.3

Total Fat: 17.1

Sodium: 656

Total Carbohydrate: 5.7

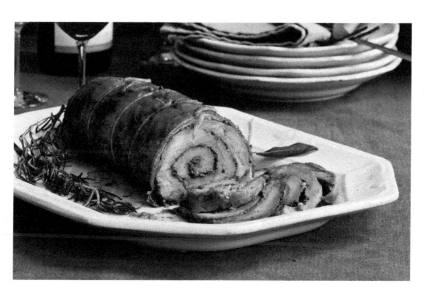

Jamaican Jerk Chicken

Serving: 6

Ingredients

- 6 skinless, boneless chicken breast halves - cut into chunks
- 4 limes, juiced
- 1 cup water
- 2 teaspoons ground allspice
- 1/2 teaspoon ground nutmeg
- 1 teaspoon salt
- 1 teaspoon brown sugar
- 2 teaspoons dried thyme
- 1 teaspoon ground ginger
- 1 1/2 teaspoons ground black pepper
- 2 tablespoons vegetable oil

- 2 onions, chopped
- 1 1/2 cups chopped green onions
- 6 cloves garlic, chopped
- 2 habanero peppers, chopped

Direction

- Marinate chicken with water and lime juice in a medium bowl. Put aside.

- In a food processor or a blender, blend the nutmeg, allspice, brown sugar, salt, thyme, black pepper, ginger and vegetable oil. Then mix in the habanero peppers, garlic, green onions, and onions until the consistency turns fine.

- Add this blend into the chicken marinade, while reserving some of the mixture to use as baste when cooking. Cover and leave, for at least 2 hours, inside the refrigerator.

- Preheat your outside grill to medium heat.

- Brush with oil the grate. Slowly cook the chicken into desired doneness; frequently baste and turn.

Nutrition Information

Calories: 221 calories;

Total Fat: 6.4

Sodium: 474

Total Carbohydrate: 13.3

Cholesterol: 68

Protein: 28.8

Japanese Style Deep Fried Chicken

Serving: 8

Ingredients

- 2 eggs, lightly beaten
- 1/2 teaspoon salt
- 1/2 teaspoon black pepper
- 1/2 teaspoon white sugar
- 1 tablespoon minced garlic
- 1 tablespoon grated fresh ginger root
- 1 tablespoon sesame oil
- 1 tablespoon soy sauce
- 1/8 teaspoon chicken bouillon granules
- 1 1/2 pounds skinless, boneless chicken breast halves - cut into 1 inch cubes

- 3 tablespoons potato starch
- 1 tablespoon rice flour
- oil for frying

Direction

- Mix together bouillon, soy sauce, sesame oil, ginger, garlic, sugar, pepper, salt and eggs in big bowl. Add chicken pieces; mix to coat then cover the bowl. Refrigerate for 30 minutes.
- Take bowl out of fridge. Add rice flour and potato starch to meat; stir well.
- Heat oil to 185°C or 365°F in a deep fryer or big skillet. Put chicken in hot oil; fry till golden brown. Working in batches, cook meat to maintain oil temperature. Place on paper towels, briefly drain; serve hot.

Nutrition Information

- Calories: 256 calories;
- Total Fat: 16.7
- Sodium: 327

- Total Carbohydrate: 4.8

- Cholesterol: 98

- Protein: 20.9

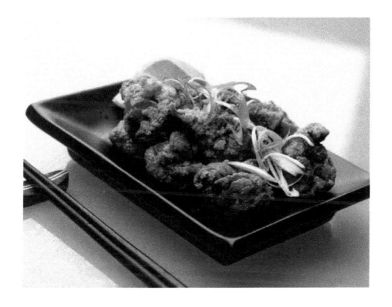

Javanese Pork Tenderloin

Serving: 8

Ingredients

- Brine:
- 1/4 cup kosher salt
- 1/4 cup brown sugar
- 3 cups warm water
- 2 (3/4 pound) pork tenderloins
- Marinade:
- 1/2 cup chunky peanut butter
- 1/4 cup sake
- 2 tablespoons soy sauce
- 2 tablespoons white wine vinegar
- 2 tablespoons honey
- 2 tablespoons peanut oil

- 2 tablespoons Thai chili paste
- 2 tablespoons Sriracha chili sauce
- 4 cloves garlic, finely minced
- 2 tablespoons fresh ginger root, finely chopped
- 1/4 cup finely chopped green onions
- 1/4 cup minced fresh cilantro (optional)

Direction

- Dissolve the brown sugar and salt in a 1/4 cup of warm water. Pour the mixture into the large resealable plastic bag together with the leftover 2 3/4 cups of water. Add the pork into the bag, and then seal it. Refrigerate the bag overnight.

- Mix the soy sauce, peanut oil, chili sauce, green onions, peanut butter, honey, ginger root, garlic, vinegar, cilantro, sake and chili paste in a small and microwavable bowl. Microwave the mixture for 30-60 seconds until the peanut butter is melted. Stir the mixture thoroughly.

- For the sauce of the cooked meat, reserve about a 1/2-3/4 cup of the peanut sauce. Refrigerate the sauce until ready to use. Transfer the remaining sauce into the resealable plastic bag. Remove the pork form brine, discarding the brine. Wash the pork and pat dry. Place the pork into the bag with the marinade. Refrigerate the bag for 8 hours or overnight.

- Set the grill over medium heat for preheating. Remove the pork from the peanut sauce marinade. Allow it to sit at room temperature for 20 minutes. Transfer the marinade into the small saucepan. Bring to a boil and boil for 3 minutes. You can add more milk to thin if the marinade is too thick.

- Oil the grill grate lightly. Place the tenderloins onto the grill. Once the pork reaches 125°F (50°C), baste it with the boiled marinade. Make sure to observe the pork after basting to avoid burning. Roll the pork around using the BBQ spatula while cooking. Grill the pork for 15 minutes until its internal temperature is 145°F (63°C). Pull the pork off from the grill and allow it to sit for 5 minutes. Slice the pork into thin rounds.

- Place the reserved sauce inside the microwave until warm. Spoon a dollop of sauce onto each of the serving plates. Top the sauce with the pork slices. Serve.

Nutrition Information

- Calories: 297 calories;

- Total Fat: 16

- Sodium: 3279

- Total Carbohydrate: 19.4

- Cholesterol: 47

- Protein: 19.4

Jerk Chicken And Pasta

Serving: 4

Ingredients

- 4 skinless, boneless chicken breast halves
- 2 teaspoons jerk paste
- 1 (12 ounce) package uncooked egg noodles
- 1 tablespoon olive oil
- 1 clove garlic, minced
- 1 cup chicken stock
- 1 tablespoon jerk paste
- 1/2 cup dry white wine
- 1/4 cup chopped fresh cilantro
- 2 limes, quartered
- salt and pepper to taste
- 1/2 cup heavy whipping cream

- 4 sprigs fresh cilantro, for garnish

Direction

- With 1/2 teaspoon jerk paste, cover each breast half, and put them in a shallow dish. For at least an hour, cover and place in a refrigerator.

- Let grill preheat on high heat. Boil lightly salted water in a large pot, add egg noodles and cook for 6 to 8 minutes until al dente, empty out the water.

- Oil grill grate lightly. Until juices are clear, grill the chicken 8-10 minutes per sides.

- In the meantime, in a large saucepan heat olive oil over medium heat, add garlic and cook for 1 minute. Add 1 tablespoon jerk paste, chicken stock, white wine, juice of 1 lime, chopped cilantro, salt, and pepper. When it boils, stir in heavy cream over low heat. For around 5 minutes, stir mixture until thick. Do not let it boil.

- Place the cooked egg noodles and toss with the cream sauce in the saucepan. Split noodles into

4 and place in serving plates put the grilled chicken on top. Garnish each plate with the juice of 1/4 lime and cilantro sprig.

Nutrition Information

- Calories: 595 calories;

- Total Fat: 25.2

- Sodium: 205

- Total Carbohydrate: 59.6

- Cholesterol: 169

- Protein: 37.3

Jollof Rice

Serving: 8

Ingredients

- 1 tablespoon olive oil
- 1 large onion, sliced
- 2 (14.5 ounce) cans stewed tomatoes
- 1/2 (6 ounce) can tomato paste
- 1 teaspoon salt
- 1/4 teaspoon black pepper
- 1/4 teaspoon cayenne pepper
- 1/2 teaspoon red pepper flakes
- 1 tablespoon Worcestershire sauce
- 1 teaspoon chopped fresh rosemary
- 2 cups water
- 1 (3 pound) whole chicken, cut into 8 pieces
- 1 cup uncooked white rice

- 1 cup diced carrots

- 1/2 pound fresh green beans, trimmed and snapped into 1 to 2 inch pieces

- 1/4 teaspoon ground nutmeg

Direction

- Put oil in a big saucepan. Cook onion in oil on medium-low heat until it's translucent.

- Mix in tomato paste and stewed tomatoes. Season using rosemary, Worcestershire sauce, red pepper flakes, cayenne pepper, black pepper, and salt. Boil, covered. Lower heat. Mix in water. Put chicken pieces. Simmer it for half an hour.

- Mix In green beans, carrots and rice. Season using nutmeg. Boil, lower heat to low. Simmer, covered, for 25-30 minutes until rice is cooked and chicken is fork-tender.

Nutrition Information

- Calories: 332 calories;

- Total Carbohydrate: 33.5

- Cholesterol: 46

- Protein: 19.8

- Total Fat: 13.4

- Sodium: 713

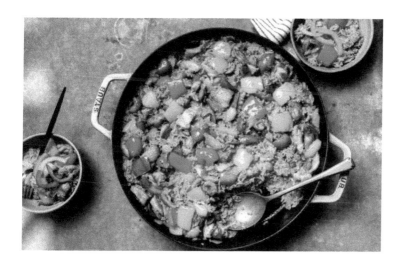

Kale Puttanesca

Serving: 4

Ingredients

- 1/2 (16 ounce) package whole-wheat angel hair pasta

- 2 tablespoons olive oil

- 1/2 large onion, sliced

- 2 cloves garlic, minced

- 1 teaspoon red pepper flakes

- 1 tablespoon drained capers

- 1 (2 ounce) can anchovy fillets, drained and quartered

- 1 cup canned diced tomatoes, undrained

- 2 cups coarsely chopped kale

- 1 (4 ounce) can sliced black olives, drained

- 1/2 cup grated Parmesan cheese, or to taste

Direction

- In a big pot, let lightly salted water boil. Put pasta and cook until al dente for 8 to 10 minutes. Drain it.

- Meanwhile, over medium-high heat, heat olive oil in a big skillet. Put pepper flakes, garlic and onions. Cook and stir for about 5 minutes until the onion has begun to turn golden brown and softened. Mix in diced tomatoes, anchovy fillets and capers. Let is simmer. Stir in kale and over medium-low heat simmer for about 10 minutes until wilted and tender.

- When the pasta is cooked and drained, mix it into puttanesca together with the black olives. Toss and use grated parmesan cheese to sprinkle. Serve.

Nutrition Information

- Calories: 361 calories;

- Total Fat: 15.6

- Sodium: 1099

- Total Carbohydrate: 41.3

- Cholesterol: 18

- Protein: 15.4

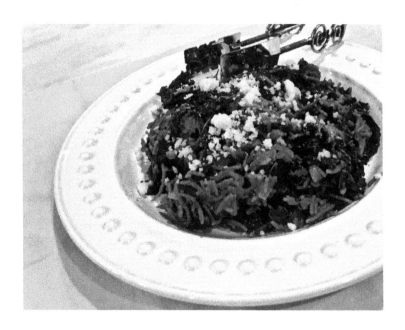

Keema (Indian Style Ground Meat)

Serving: 4

Ingredients

- 1 1/2 pounds ground lamb
- 1 onion, finely chopped
- 2 cloves garlic, minced
- 2 tablespoons garam masala
- 1 teaspoon salt
- 4 teaspoons tomato paste
- 3/4 cup beef broth

Direction

Cook the ground lamb in a large heavy skillet over medium heat until it turns brown evenly. Use a wooden spoon to break it apart while cooking until it is crumbled. Place the cooked lamb into a bowl, then drain off all but

93

retain a tablespoon of fat. Sauté the onion for 5 minutes until it is translucent and soft. Mix in the garlic, sauté for a minute. Stir in salt and garam masala and cook for a minute. Place the browned lamb back into the pan, then stir in beef broth and tomato paste. Turn down the heat and simmer until the liquid evaporates and the meat is completely cooked through, about 10 - 15 minutes.

Nutrition Information

- Calories: 513 calories;
- Total Fat: 40.7
- Sodium: 885
- Total Carbohydrate: 6.4
- Cholesterol: 124
- Protein: 29.6

Spicy Curry Chicken

Serving: 6

Ingredients

- 2 (14 ounce) cans coconut milk

- 2 tablespoons green curry paste

- 2/3 cup chicken broth

- 1 (8 ounce) can sliced water chestnuts, drained

- 1 (8 ounce) can sliced bamboo shoots, drained

- 1 green bell pepper, cut into 1 inch pieces

- 1 cup sliced fresh mushrooms

- 3 boneless skinless chicken breasts, cut into 1 inch pieces

- 3 tablespoons fish sauce

- 1/4 cup chopped fresh basil

Direction

- In a large saucepan, whisk together curry paste and coconut milk over medium heat. Let to simmer for five minutes.

- Mix in chicken, mushrooms, bell pepper, bamboo shoots, water chestnuts and chicken broth. Season with basil and fish sauce. Let simmer for about ten minutes longer or until the chicken is cooked but still tender.

Nutrition Information

- Calories: 416 calories;

- Protein: 29.1

- Total Fat: 33.4

- Sodium: 717

- Total Carbohydrate: 12.1

- Cholesterol: 61

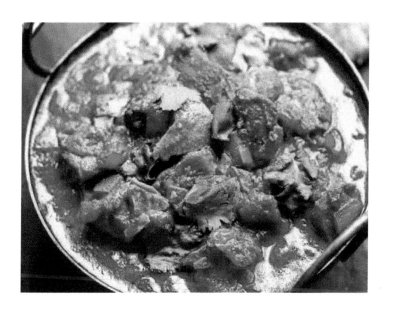

Lamb For Lovers

Serving: 4

Ingredients

2 tablespoons olive oil

2 (7 bone) racks of lamb, trimmed, fat reserved

salt and pepper to taste

4 cloves garlic, minced

1 large onion, diced

4 carrots, diced

1 cup celery tops

1 cup port wine

1 cup red wine

1 (14.5 ounce) can low-sodium chicken broth

5 sprigs fresh spearmint

3 sprigs fresh rosemary

1 cup mint apple jelly

2 tablespoons olive oil

salt and pepper to taste

1 tablespoon garlic, minced

1/4 cup panko bread crumbs

2 tablespoons olive oil

4 sprigs fresh mint

Direction

Making Demi-Glace: In a medium skillet, heat two tablespoons of olive oil on medium heat and then place in trimmings from the lamb. Season with pepper and salt, then brown the fat, lower the heat and add chicken broth, red wine, port, celery leaves, carrots, onion and 4 cloves minced garlic. Place mixture into a slow cooker and let it simmer for 8 hours or overnight on Low.

Over medium-low heat, strain the mixture from slow cooker into saucepan. Stir in mint jelly, rosemary and spearmint. Simmer while adding extra broth, wine or port as needed, until the mixture leaves behind a coating like that of a syrup on the back of a spoon, then strain again and keep it warm as the lamb roasts.

Roasting the Lamb: Put an oven-proof skillet or a cast iron in an oven and then preheat to 230 degrees C (450 degrees F). Rub the lamb with garlic, pepper, salt and two tablespoons of olive oil, then coat with the panko bread crumbs.

Gently take out the heated skillet from oven. Heat two tablespoons of olive oil in skillet and then sear the lamb on each side. Place skillet containing the lamb back into the oven and continue to cook for 5 to 10 minutes, until the internal temperature is 63 degrees C (145 degrees F).

Place a little amount of demi-glace onto a platter and then arrange the lamb crisscrossed. Drizzle with additional demi-glace and stud with fresh mint. Serve.

Nutrition Information

Calories: 1246 calories;

Cholesterol: 192

Protein: 45.3

Total Fat: 79.4

Sodium: 422

Total Carbohydrate: 68.4

Lemon Chicken II

Serving: 6

Ingredients

- 3 pounds boneless chicken breasts, cut into 2-inch pieces
- 1 tablespoon dry sherry
- 1 tablespoon soy sauce
- 1/2 teaspoon salt
- 2 eggs
- 2 cups vegetable oil
- 1/4 cup cornstarch
- 1/2 teaspoon baking powder
- 1/3 cup white sugar
- 1 tablespoon cornstarch
- 1 cup chicken broth

- 1 tablespoon lemon juice

- 1 teaspoon salt

- 1 lemon, sliced

- 2 tablespoons vegetable oil

Direction

- Combine half a teaspoon of salt, chicken pieces, soy sauce, and sherry in a large bowl. Stir well, then cover with lid or plastic wrap and refrigerate. Leave to marinade for 15 to 20 minutes.

- Mix baking powder and a quarter cup of cornstarch in a small bowl. To make the batter, add eggs into the mixture. Coat each piece of chicken then set aside.

- Heat two cups of oil in a wok or large saucepan until the oil temperature reaches 350°F or 175°C. Fry the chicken until brown. Work in batches. Transfer the cooked pieces on a plate covered with paper towels.

- Whisk together a teaspoon of salt, broth, lemon juice, sugar, and a tablespoon of cornstarch in a medium-sized bowl. Add in lemon slices into the mixture. In a small skillet, heat up two tablespoons of oil. Pour in the lemon sauce mixture; cook and stir until the sauce becomes clear. Dress the fried chicken with the sauce before serving.

Nutrition Information

Calories: 490 calories;

Total Fat: 20.8

Sodium: 932

Total Carbohydrate: 20.9

Cholesterol: 200

Protein: 53.4

Linguine All'Aragosta (Lobster Linguine)

Serving: 4

Ingredients

- 2 (5 ounce) uncooked lobster tails

- 1/4 cup unsalted butter, cubed

- 3 scallions, white parts only, minced

- 1 1/2 tablespoons minced garlic

- 8 Roma tomatoes, crushed (concasse)

- 1 tablespoon chili powder

- 1 1/2 teaspoons dried basil

- 1 cup Chablis wine

- 1 (16 ounce) package linguine pasta

- 1/4 cup light cream

- 1 scallion, green part only, thinly sliced

- 1 pinch sea salt and ground black pepper to taste

- 2 tablespoons grated Parmesan cheese (optional)

Direction

- In a saucepan, put a steamer insert in and fill with water to right beneath the streamer's bottom. Put a cover on and boil the water over high heat. Add lobster tails, cover again and steam for 10 minutes until no longer opaque in the middle. Separate the meat from shell and slice into bite-sized chunks.

- In a big frying pan over medium heat, melt butter. Add garlic and scallion whites, stir and cook for 1-2 minutes until fragrant. Add basil, chili powder, and tomatoes. Cook for 2-3 minutes until the tomatoes are slightly tender. Add wine; lower the heat to medium-low. Cook the sauce without a cover on, tossing sometimes for 30 minutes until the wine is vaporized.

- Boil a big pot of lightly salted water. Cook linguine once boiling for 11 minutes until soft but firm to the bite. Strain.

- Lower the heat under the sauce. Add scallion greens, cream and lobster, cook for 5-10 minutes until the consistency reaches the thickness you want. Use pepper and sea salt to season. Add pasta in batches, mixing well to coat after each adding. Use Parmesan cheese to sprinkle on top.

Nutrition Information

- Calories: 694 calories;

- Cholesterol: 85

- Protein: 29.5

- Total Fat: 20

- Sodium: 609

- Total Carbohydrate: 93.3

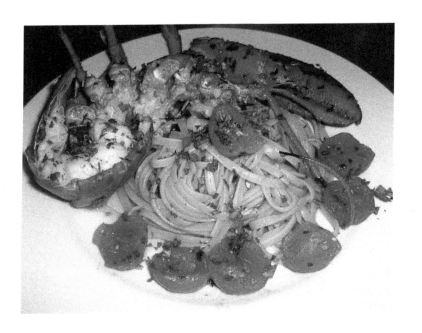

Lobster Fricassee

Serving: 4

Ingredients

- 1/2 cup finely chopped carrot
- 1/2 cup chopped celery
- 1/2 cup chopped onion
- 2 cups dry white wine
- 2 (1 1/2 pound) whole lobsters
- 2 tablespoons brandy
- 1/2 cup heavy cream
- 2 tablespoons unsalted butter

Direction

- Mix white wine, onion, celery, and carrot together in a big frying pan. Boil it. Put lobsters, put a cover on, and cook for 8 minutes until the lobsters are shiny red. Take the lobsters out from the sauce and let it cool down.

- Once the lobsters are cool enough to touch, slice each one in two lengthwise. Separate the meat from the claws and shell, save it and do not break the shell.

- Dispose the tomalley if you want. Cut each tail into 4 medallions and put aside.

- Keep simmering the vegetables and wine in the frying pan for 10 minutes until there is half of the liquid left. Put the shell back to the sauce and mix in the brandy. Simmer for 5 minutes. Use a mesh strainer or a sieve to filter the stock through into a saucepan. Mix in the heavy cream and cook on medium heat for 10 minutes until firm. Mix in the butter just until melted. Put lobster meat in the sauce and cook over low heat until cooked through.

Nutrition Information

Calories: 602 calories;

Total Fat: 19.9

Sodium: 1051

Total Carbohydrate: 9.7

Cholesterol: 379

Protein: 65.3

Macadamia Crusted Sea Bass With Mango Cream Sauce

Serving: 4

Ingredients

- 1/2 mango - peeled, seeded and diced
- 1/2 cup heavy cream
- 1 teaspoon lemon juice
- 1/2 cup chopped macadamia nuts
- 1/4 cup seasoned bread crumbs
- 1 teaspoon olive oil
- 1/2 teaspoon black pepper
- 1 pinch red pepper flakes
- 1 pound fresh sea bass
- salt and ground black pepper to taste

- 2 cloves minced garlic

- 1 tablespoon extra virgin olive oil

Direction

- Mix red pepper flakes, black pepper, 1 teaspoon of olive oil, bread crumbs, and macadamia nuts together in a food processor. Blend until creamy. Start preheating the oven to 350°F (175°C).

- Mix lemon juice, cream, and mango together over medium heat in a small saucepan. Boil it, lower the heat, and simmer it until thickened.

- Use black pepper and salt to season the fish. In a big frying pan, heat 1 tablespoon of olive oil and mash garlic over medium heat. Sear both sides of the sea bass and take away from heat.

- Put the fish in the preheated oven and roast until cooked through. Use macadamia crust to cover the sea bass and put it back to the oven until the crusts turn brown. Put the mango cream sauce on top.

Nutrition Information

- Calories: 423 calories;

- Total Fat: 31.1

- Sodium: 222

- Total Carbohydrate: 13.6

- Cholesterol: 87

- Protein: 24.2

Mahi Mahi With Onions And Mushrooms

Serving: 4

Ingredients

2 tablespoons olive oil

3 small onions, chopped

4 cloves garlic, minced

5 button mushrooms, sliced

1 1/2 pounds mahi mahi

salt and pepper to taste

1/4 cup white cooking wine

1 tablespoon fresh lemon juice

1 teaspoon cornstarch

2 tablespoons water

Direction

- Pour olive oil into a big skillet. At medium heat, heat the oil. Insert the garlic, mushrooms and onions, cooking until the onions become translucent. Slice the fillets up fish up into fillets, about 3 inches long. On top of the garlic, mushrooms and onions, set the mahi-mahi fillets down. Add pepper and salt to the fillet's first side to your liking. Pour in lemon juice and white cooking wine. Leave it cooking with the cover on for 4-5 minutes. After turning the fillets over, add pepper and salt onto the second side to your liking. Leave it cooking until the flesh starts flaking with ease, about another 4-5 minutes. Transfer the fish along onto a heated plate. Maintain the warmth until the sauce is done. Inside of the skillet with cooking wine, garlic, mushrooms and onion, turn the heat up to medium-high. Boil. Mix 2 tablespoons of water with corn-starch until dissolved, stirring this into the skillet. Keep stirring the sauce consistently until the sauce is at personal preference of consistency. Before serving at once, empty the sauce out atop the mahi-mahi fillets.

Nutrition Information

- Calories: 251 calories;

- Total Fat: 8.1

- Sodium: 155

- Total Carbohydrate: 8

- Cholesterol: 124

- Protein: 33

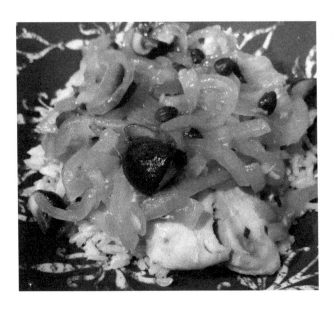

Malaysian Beef Rendang

Serving: 6

Ingredients

- 3/8 pound shallots

- 3 cloves garlic

- 15 dried red chile peppers

- 5 slices fresh ginger root

- 5 lemon grass, chopped

- 2 teaspoons coriander seeds

- 2 teaspoons fennel seeds

- 2 teaspoons cumin seeds

- 1 pinch grated nutmeg

- 1 tablespoon vegetable oil

- 1 1/4 pounds beef stew meat, cut into 1 inch cubes

- 1 1/2 tablespoons white sugar

- 2 cups shredded coconut

- 5 whole cloves

- 1 cinnamon stick

- 1 2/3 cups coconut milk

- 7/8 cup water

- salt to taste

Direction

- In a dry wok, heat the coconut, mixing constantly till golden brown. Reserve to cool down.

- Blend the lemon grass, ginger, chilies, garlic and shallots using a food processor or a blender to a thick paste.

- Grind the nutmeg, cumin, fennel and coriander.

- Fry the shallot paste in a small amount of oil using the wok for a several minutes. Put the nutmeg, cumin, fennel and ground coriander;

cook for 3 to 4 minutes, mixing constantly. Put beef; over medium heat cook till meat is browned for 3 to 4 minutes longer.

- Mix in water, coconut milk, cinnamon stick, cloves, coconut and sugar. Boil, reduce heat, and allow to simmer for an hour till the meat is tender and most of the liquid has gone. Put salt to taste.

Nutrition Information

- Calories: 654 calories;

- Total Carbohydrate: 24.9

- Cholesterol: 63

- Protein: 22.3

- Total Fat: 54.5

- Sodium: 83

Maple Glazed Chipotle Goat Cheese Lamb Burgers

Serving: 4

Ingredients

1 head garlic

1 pound ground lamb

6 ounces soft goat cheese

6 tablespoons minced chipotle peppers in adobo sauce

2 sprigs chopped fresh rosemary

2 tablespoons maple syrup

1 1/2 teaspoons salt

1/2 teaspoon cracked black pepper

1 tablespoon olive oil

2 tablespoons maple syrup

4 ciabatta buns, split and toasted

Direction

- Set an oven to 150°C (300°F). Remove the top of the head of garlic and put on a small, oven-safe dish.

- Bake the garlic in the prepared oven for about an hour until the cloves turn golden brown and soft. Take away from the oven, and allow to cool. In a mixing bowl, squeeze the roasted garlic when it is cool enough to handle. Mix thoroughly pepper, salt, 2 tablespoons of maple syrup, rosemary, chipotle peppers, goat cheese, and the lamb. Shape into 4 patties.

- In a large skillet, heat the olive oil on medium-high. Sear the lamb patties for 1 minute per side, then turn the heat down to medium-low, and keep on cooking for around 2 minutes on each side for medium-well to the desired doneness. Around a minute before the patties are done, add in the remaining 2 tablespoons of maple syrup; let it glaze and thicken the burgers. Serve together with toasted ciabatta buns.

Nutrition Information

- Calories: 609 calories;

- Total Fat: 33.7

- Sodium: 1482

- Total Carbohydrate: 42

- Cholesterol: 110

- Protein: 33.5

Maple Garlic Marinated Pork Tenderloin

Serving: 6

Ingredients

2 tablespoons Dijon mustard

1 teaspoon sesame oil

3 cloves garlic, minced

fresh ground black pepper to taste

1 cup maple syrup

1 1/2 pounds pork tenderloin

Direction

Mix together the maple syrup, pepper, garlic, sesame oil and mustard. In a shallow dish, put the pork and coat it with the marinade thoroughly. Put cover and let it chill in the fridge for a minimum of 8 hours or overnight.

Set the grill to preheat to medium-low heat.

Take out the pork from the marinade and put aside. Move the leftover marinade to a small saucepan and let it cook for 5 minutes on the stove on medium-low heat.

Brush oil on the grate and put the meat on the grate. Grill the pork and baste it with the reserved marinade for about 15-25 minutes or until the inside has no visible pink color. Do not use high temperatures as the marinade will burn.

Nutrition Information

- Calories: 288 calories;
- Total Fat: 4.9
- Sodium: 189
- Total Carbohydrate: 36.8
- Cholesterol: 74
- Protein: 23.5

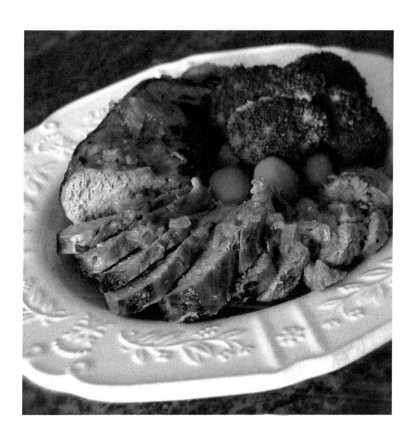

Mediterranean Lemon Chicken

Serving: 6

Ingredients

- 1 lemon

- 2 teaspoons dried oregano

- 3 cloves garlic, minced

- 1 tablespoon olive oil

- 1/4 teaspoon salt

- 1/4 teaspoon ground black pepper

- 6 chicken legs

Direction

- Set the oven to 425°F or 220°C for preheating.

- In a 9x13-inches baking dish, grate the peel from the lemon half. Squeeze the juice out from the lemon, about 1/4 cup of juice, and add it into the peel together with the pepper, oil, oregano, salt, and garlic. Stir the mixture until well blended.

- Remove and discard the skin from the chicken pieces. Coat the lemon mixture all over the chicken pieces. Arrange the chicken into the baking dish, bone-side up. Cover the dish and bake the chicken for 20 minutes. Flip the chicken and baste.

- Adjust the heat to 400°F or 205°C. Bake the chicken while uncovered for 30 more minutes, basting the chicken every 10 minutes. Serve the chicken together with its pan juices.

Nutrition Information

- Calories: 241 calories;

- Total Fat: 11.8

- Sodium: 200

- Total Carbohydrate: 2.8

- Cholesterol: 105

Mediterranean Salmon

Serving: 4

Ingredients

1/2 cup olive oil

1/4 cup balsamic vinegar

4 cloves garlic, pressed

4 (3 ounce) fillets salmon

1 tablespoon chopped fresh cilantro

1 tablespoon chopped fresh basil

1 1/2 teaspoons garlic salt

Direction

In a small bowl, combine together the balsamic vinegar and olive oil. Spread salmon fillets onto a shallow baking dish. Brush garlic over the fillets, and then spread the oil and vinegar on top of them flipping once to coat. Season with garlic salt, basil, and cilantro. Save to marinate for ten minutes.

Preheat the oven's broiler.

Put salmon approximately 6 inches away from the heat and broil for about 15 minutes, flipping once, or until fish is browned on each side and flaked easily with a fork. Baste often with sauce from the pan.

Nutrition Information

- Calories: 391 calories;

- Sodium: 725

- Total Carbohydrate: 3.6

- Cholesterol: 42

- Protein: 15

- Total Fat: 35.2

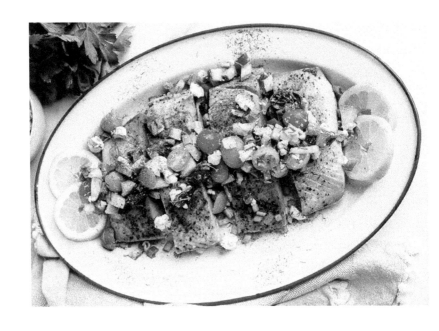

Mediterranean Seafood Medley

Serving: 6

Ingredients

- 20 baby squid (tubes and tentacles), cleaned
- 3 cups milk
- 2 tablespoons extra-virgin olive oil
- 8 cloves garlic, minced
- 2 small onions, chopped
- 2 large carrots, chopped
- 2 tomatoes, chopped
- 1 small fennel bulb, diced
- 1/2 cup tomato paste
- 1 cup dry white wine
- 3 cups chicken stock

- 1/2 bunch fresh parsley
- 1/2 bunch fresh tarragon
- 1/2 bunch fresh thyme
- 2 bay leaves
- 1 teaspoon black peppercorns
- 1 tablespoon loosely packed saffron threads
- 2 tablespoons extra-virgin olive oil
- 6 cloves garlic, minced
- 1/2 cup oil-packed sun-dried tomatoes, drained and cut into strips
- 6 baby fennel bulbs, halved
- 1/2 bunch fresh thyme, chopped
- 10 fresh oysters in shells, well scrubbed
- 20 littleneck clams
- 20 fresh mussels
- 6 (6 ounce) fillets fresh sea bass
- salt and pepper to taste
- 2 tablespoons extra-virgin olive oil

- 6 sprigs parsley, for garnish

Direction

In milk, soak squid for 1-5 hours, preferably longer. When squid finishes soaking, drain then discard milk.

In a big pot, heat 2 tablespoons olive oil on medium heat. Mix in diced fennel, tomatoes, carrots, onions, and garlic. Sauté for about 10 minutes until veggies soften. Mix in tomato paste then cook for additional 10 minutes. Put in wine, increase heat up to high. When it boils, add saffron, peppercorns, bay leaves, thyme, tarragon, parsley, and chicken stock. Boil again, reduce heat down to medium, then simmer until all liquid reduces to one and a half cups for about 15 minutes. Strain liquid out. Discard solids.

In a big pot, heat 2 tablespoons olive oil on medium heat. Mix in garlic, cooking for about 45 seconds until fragrant. Add fennel and sun-dried tomatoes. Cook for about 2 minutes. Pour in strained saffron broth and the chopped thyme. Bring heat up to medium-high and boil. Put oysters on fennel. Cover then cook for a minute. Set mussels and clams in the pot. Cover and cook for about 4 minutes until shellfish starts to open. Mix in strained squid, cover again, and cook until squid firms for 1 minute.

As shellfish cooks, season sea bass fillets with pepper and salt. In a big skillet, heat leftover 2 tablespoons olive oil on medium-high heat. Put fish in a skillet with the skin-side down. Cover then cook until fish's flesh is firm and not translucent and skin is crispy.

Pour fennel-seafood mixture on a serving platter. Put sea bass fillets on it. Garnish with parsley sprigs. Serve.

Nutrition Information

Calories: 641 calories;

Total Fat: 25.8

Sodium: 897

Total Carbohydrate: 35.8

Cholesterol: 313

Protein: 60.2

Millet Mung Bean Main Dish

Serving: 12

Ingredients

- 9 cups water, divided
- 2 cups dried mung beans
- 2 1/2 cups millet
- 1 tablespoon vegetable oil
- 1 large onion, chopped
- 1 green bell pepper, chopped
- 1 stalk celery, chopped
- 1 carrot, shredded, or more to taste
- 2/3 bunch chopped flat-leaf parsley
- 2 cloves garlic, minced
- 1 (1 inch) piece fresh ginger, grated

- 2 teaspoons dried basil, or more to taste
- 1 teaspoon dried oregano
- 1 teaspoon ground cumin
- 1 teaspoon curry powder
- 1/2 teaspoon cayenne pepper
- 2 cups chopped tomatoes
- 2 teaspoons salt
- ground black pepper to taste
- 2 cups shredded sharp Cheddar cheese

Direction

Boil the mung beans and 4 cups of water in a pot. Put cover and lower the heat to medium-low, then simmer for 45-60 minutes, until the beans become tender.

In another pot, boil the millet and 5 cups of water. Put cover and lower the heat to medium-low, then simmer for 10-20 minutes, until the millet becomes tender and the water has been absorbed.

In a fry pan, heat the oil on medium heat. Let cook and stir the cayenne pepper, curry powder, cumin, oregano, basil, ginger, garlic, parsley, carrot, celery, green bell pepper and onion for 5-10 minutes, until the veggies turn a bit tender. Mix the pepper, salt and tomatoes into the veggie mixture.

Stir the Cheddar cheese, millet and mung beans into the veggie mixture, then let it cook while stirring for 2-3 minutes, until the cheese melts.

Nutrition Information

- Calories: 381 calories;
- Total Carbohydrate: 55.2
- Cholesterol: 20
- Protein: 18.8
- Total Fat: 9.9
- Sodium: 536

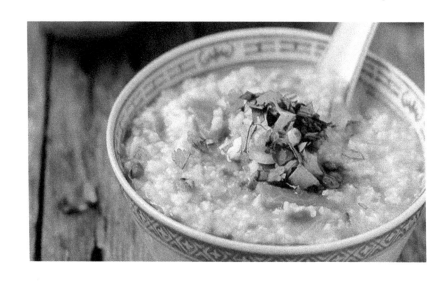

THANK YOU

Thank you for choosing *Healthy Recipes for Beginners Lunch* for improving your cooking skills! I hope you enjoyed making the recipes as much as tasting them! If you're interested in learning new recipes and new meals to cook, go and check out the other books of the series.